Purpose of AdventureBC:

Adventure BC aims to capture British Columbia (BC) fun and share it with the world. Our mandate is to showcase the diversity of people, countries, cultures exploring what B.C. offers. We seach out sneak peeks to the adventurous activities that can be found in this amazing Province. We believe that people should be proactive in safeguarding their health and use this platform to encourage people to get outdoors and live a healthy active lifestyle.

AdventureBC also strives to motivate people through social media, public marketing, photos, and writings. We are passionate about inspiring people to actively pursue their dreams and to live life to its fullest. As we strive to drive tourism, we also look to make companies better, promote exciting locations and give people an insight into the best travel experiences possible.

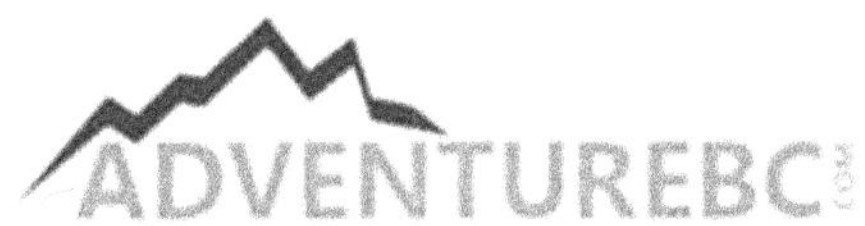

Share Your Adventure & Get a Free T-Shirt

AdventureBC is dedicated to showcasing people, outdoor sports, product & gear reviews and activities related adventure/ecotourism businesses. We look forward to your articles on outdoor events and activities and want to hear about your super fun adventures in British Columbia.

Let Us Share Your Story to the world, and we will send you a FREE T-Shirt!

Submission Guidelines

Present an original, clear, and exciting adventure and not merely a topic or idea. Our features generally range from 500 to 1,000 words in length. We generally feature: destinations pieces, news, advice for adventurous travelers, and/or reviews/evaluations of outdoor gear and equipment.

Please proofread your article before making your submission.

Each article should include a short biography of the author.

We reserve the right to edit all submissions before posting.

Image Guidelines

Your submission must include two or three relevant images.

Image Format

Photos must be submitted separately and be a minimum of 1024 pixels wide in jpg format.

Do not embed photos into the article; they will not be accepted.

Articles without a photo will not be published. All photos must include photo credits.

Contents

Introduction

The world has seen quite a number of revolutions, and from time to time we make modifications that are so significant that they create a ripple effect that forces us to change the way we think, act and do things. In the last decade or so, the world has seen another shift; and we have seen an increased focus on health and fitness. The daily ads and scientific findings are quick to point out the correlation between a healthy lifestyle and happiness and longevity. We are repeatedly shown the benefits of exercise and the importance of having balanced meals and there is a push now than ever to take our lives into our own hands.

This book is designed to assist you on your journey to becoming a better healthier person. It will provide tips, tricks and practical advice on how to stay fit and healthy in these modern times. The truth is there are many myths and misconceptions about health that need to be debunked and staying fit and healthy does not have to be a constant struggle. This book will show you how to make health and fitness an integral part of your lifestyle and will how to move away from the idea that staying fit and healthy is a temporary summer craze.

Read on and find out more about how you can live, breathe, eat, move and think healthier.

Healthy Living for a Better You

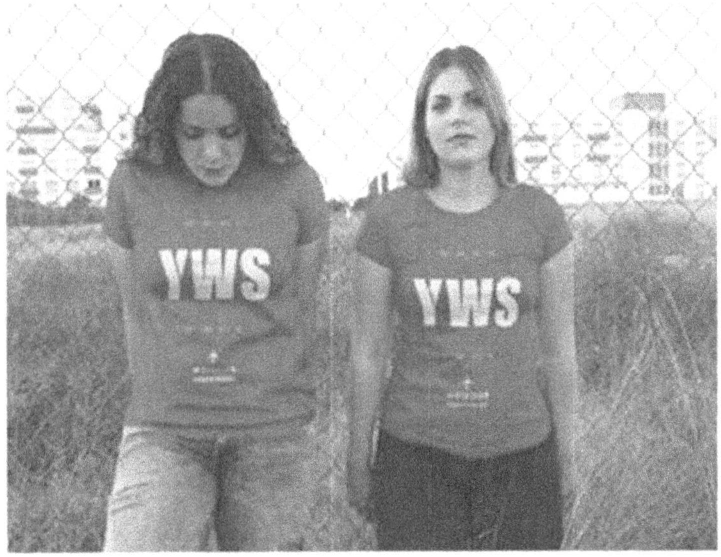

Nobody really holds the key to life; it is as elusive as the fabled fountain of youth. Nevertheless, we can control the quality of our lives and maintaining a healthy lifestyle is one of the ways in which we can contribute to our longevity.

So what exactly is a healthy lifestyle? A healthy lifestyle speaks to a way of living that lowers the risk of being seriously ill or dying early. Sure, life is a gamble, and not all diseases are preventable, but some, particularly certain lifestyle diseases such as hypertension, coronary heart disease and certain cancers can be avoided. In fact, there is scientific evidence to suggest that certain types of behavior or lifestyles contribute to the development of non-communicable diseases and early death.

It is therefore in our best interest to safeguard our health at every stage of our lives and we should move away from the ill-conceived idea that being healthy is just about avoiding diseases because that is only one aspect of it. Being healthy is about making a conscious effort to safeguard one's physical, mental and social well-being. A healthy person will be physically and mentally alert and they will more than likely be a pleasure to be around.

Key Tips to Eating Healthy

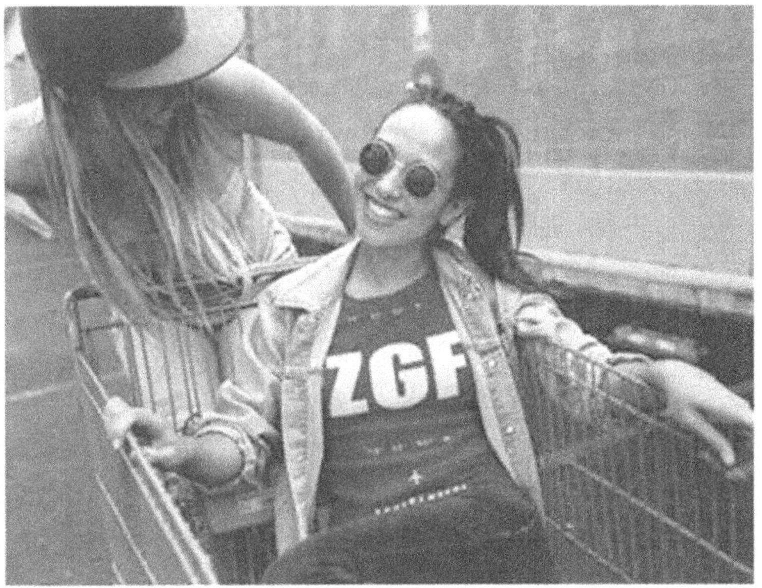

EAT A BALANCED DIET

This may sound rather clichéd but it is true; we are what we eat. All of us relieve our hunger pangs daily by grabbing a bite but not all of us make a conscious note of what we eat and even more of us fail in the balancing act. In fact, some of us would not know what a balanced meal is even if it insisted on reversing roles and biting us. Nevertheless, it is never too late to do something about it and you most certainly can. Always bear in mind that there are 6 main food groups; fruits, vegetable, protein food, grains, carbohydrates and dairy.

In order to ensure that you are on the right path, you may consider the following rule of the thumb; half of your daily diet should be fruits and vegetables. Protein foods include meat (lean meat is recommended), seafood, eggs, nut, peas, beans and soy. It is recommended that women should have at least 5 ½ ounces per day while men should eat at least 6 ½ ounces and vegetarians should consume at least 8 ounces of seafood derived protein per week. Women over 30 should consume 5 ounces per day and men over 50 should limit their intake to 6 ounces per day.

Make it a habit of eating whole grains and calcium fortified dairy products in moderation is also advised and it is important to note that food such as cream cheese, butter and cream are not good sources of dairy. A balanced diet as the name suggests should have all the food groups in the correct proportion. Be sure to drink lots of water at intervals but do not drink while you eat and limit sugar in your diet (this will be hard at first because sugar is addictive but it can be done if you are determined enough). You owe it to your body and your loved ones because a healthy diet could save you trips to the doctor and it is one of the surest ways of lengthening your life span.

A Practical Guide for Planning Your Meals:

In a nutshell, the tips I'm giving here whittle down to the time-tested strategy of balance, variety, and moderation. Here are few things you should consider:

1.   Go For Variety
According to food experts, you need more than 40 different nutrients for good health and no one food provides them all. Therefore, you need to choose a variety of nutrient-dense foods that include fruits and vegetables, whole grain, meat; poultry; dairy products; fish and other protein foods in order to get a variety of nutrients.

2.   Balanced Menu
If you are in the habit of eating food high in carbohydrates, fat or sugar, then make a conscious effort to reduce your intake and include all the other food groups. If you miss out any food group

one day, make up for it the next day but your overall menu in a week should constitute a healthy diet.

3. Eat according to your eating pattern

While some foods are more nutritious than others, try to move away from the tendency of labelling some foods 'good' and others 'bad' because in reality eating in moderation is key. So you do not need to feel guilty when you eat fried stuff, potato chips, chocolates, cookies, cakes; fast foods. The most important thing is to eat them in moderation and eat other foods that will provide the balance and variety.

4. Pin On Plenty of Whole Grains, Fruits & Vegetables

You should aim to get 6-11 servings from the food group that contains bread, rice, pasta and cereal, of which 3 servings should be whole grains.

P/S: 1 serving = 1 piece or 4 oz

P/S: Whole grains are foods such as oatmeal, whole-wheat bread/pasta, brown rice and barley

Eat 2-4 servings of fruits and 3-5 servings of vegetables

P/S: 1 serving of fruit = 1 piece or 4 oz; 1 serving of vegetable = 6 oz

5. Go for Moderate Portions

What's a moderate portion? The term moderate can be somewhat objective but here is an example that you may find helpful. In the case of cooked meat, the portion you should eat is 3 oz which is roughly the same size as a deck of playing cards. It is a good idea to first determine your daily intake and plan your meals accordingly but the simple rule of thumb is to be reasonable in your approach. Stop eating when you're full. Don't overeat.

6. Don't Totally Eliminate Certain Foods

This may come as a shock to you but you do not need to take the extremist approach to healthy eating in order to eat healthy. So, don't permanently cut certain foods out of your diet simply because they are perceived as "bad. Instead simply reduce the intake of these "bad" foods. That means if you love ice cream; cakes or pizzas, you don't have to give them up; just eat them less often and eat moderate or smaller portions.

7. Adhere To Regular Meals

Regular meals mean breakfast, lunch and dinner. Don't skip these 3 regular meals as skipping them could make you more hungry and will cause you to resort to over-eating. Find healthy snacks if you are in the habit of snacking provided you don't snack so much that you can't eat your regular meals.

8. "Feast" At Lunch Time

Whenever possible, eat your main meal at lunch and a light meal at dinner. This is a healthier way to eat and good for your body's digestive system.

9. Hydration

Drink plenty of water to keep your body hydrated.

Use these tips to make gradual changes in your menu. Don't suddenly change overnight beause you will not be able to cope due to the overwhelming effect and it may hamper your goal of eating healthily. Just start with small changes; you'd be amazed how they add up to become positive, permanent eating habits.

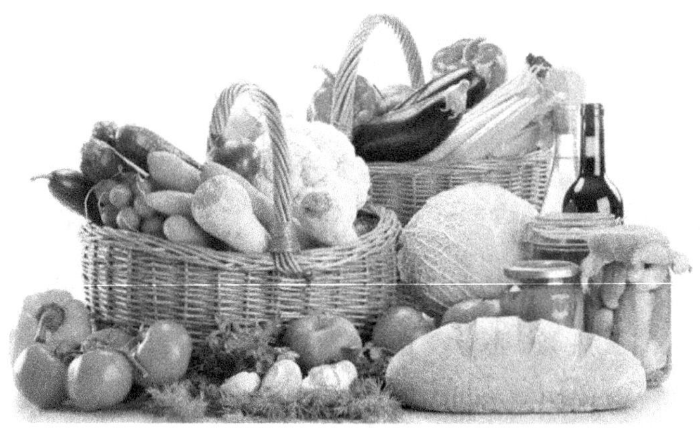

10 Great Foods That Will Help You to Get Fit and Healthy

When it comes to food, opinions vary and with the rise of health consciousness, we have seen a proliferation of food gurus, here, there and just about everywhere. In fact, many people tell us that we should not be eating any carbohydrates. They tell us that certain foods are bad and food like fat have been given a bad rap. Nevertheless, I'm here to tell you that you can eat both fat and carbohydrates. Now here's the kicker; make sure the kind of carbohydrates and fat you eat are the good ones and you should complement your diet with high-quality protein.

Here, I'm going to list some good foods that contain good fats, good carbohydrates, and good proteins. They are all high quality and will help your body improve.

1. Sardines:

Sardines as a source of protein and Omega 3 fats is underrated. Heck, they are even better than salmon in this regard. Add some to your diet and you will start building a leaner body along with a number of other benefits.

2. Quinoa:

This amino-acid rich grain is one of the few plant proteins that offer a complete protein. It is also a good source of carbohydrates. Though it is considered a grain, it is more related to spinach or Swiss chard. It is also rich in other vital minerals such as such as magnesium and manganese.

3. Goat's milk:

While most people drink cow's milk, it is goat's milk that more closely matches our own. It is more digestible and for those with allergies to cow's milk, it makes a good alternative. Goat's milk is loaded with the amino acid tryptophan as well as calcium.

4. Brown rice:

Brown rice and white rice come from the same source. The process that destroys much of the nutrients that converts rice to its white color is preserved in brown rice. Only the outermost hull is removed from the rice grain, keeping the brown rice intact. Brown rice has a good source of manganese as well as selenium and magnesium. The carbohydrates will help you maintain good energy levels throughout the day.

6. Sweet potatoes:

These foods are high in beta-carotene which is converted into

Vitamin A by your body. Studies have shown Vitamin A to be helpful in fighting cancer. Sweet potatoes are low in calories and high in fiber. They are also another source of good carbohydrates.

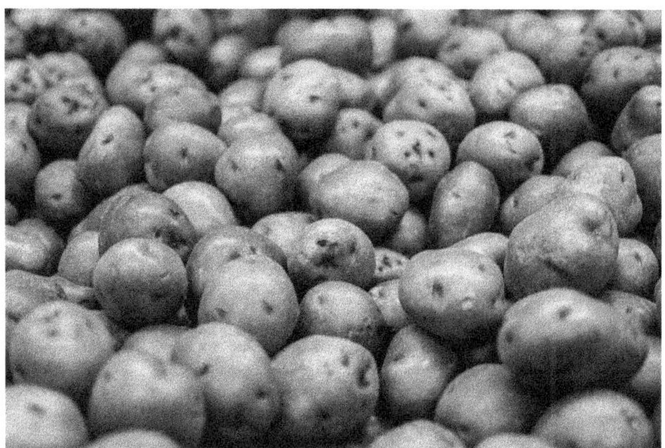
Sweet potatoes are a rich source of beta-carotene

7. Broccoli:
This vegetable contains a lot of fiber and phytonutrients. Phytonutrients contain compounds that may prevent cancer.

8. Apple:
An excellent source of pectin, which helps lower cholesterol and blood glucose. There are other excellent nutrients in an apple. It's also a great source of fast carbohydrates prior to a workout. No wonder people have been saying "An apple a day will keep the doctor away" because there is indeed some truth in it.

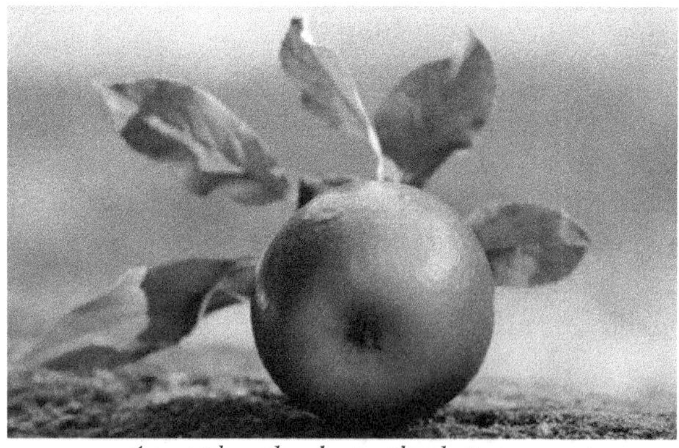
An apple a day keeps the doctor away

9. Blueberries:

This is yet another great source of phytonutrients and Vitamin C. Some studies have shown that blueberries are great in helping improve short- term memory loss.

10. Almonds:

This is one of of the best plant sources of protein. Almond contain monounsaturated fats that are actually good for us and as far as nuts are concerned, these have the highest source of calcium.

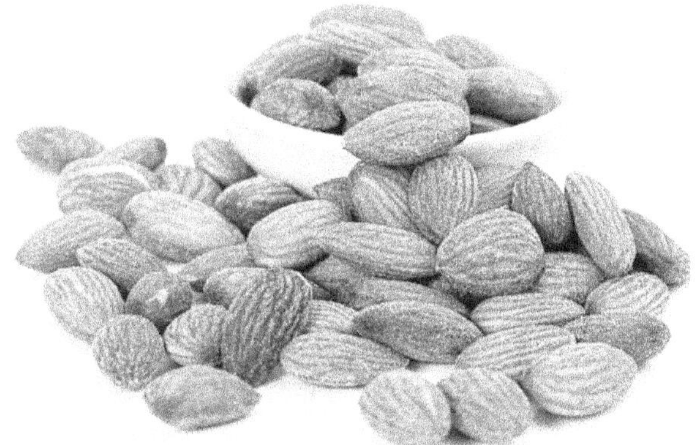

Roasted Almond Seeds

11. Spinach:

Whenever I think of spinach, I think of Popeye the Sailor. These are great in Vitamin A, C, and Folate. It also contains iron, calcium, Vitamin B-6, riboflavin, and magnesium. All of these help to promote healthy skin and hair. No wonder Popeye always said after he ate his spinach, "I'm strong to the finish because I eats me spinach..."

Getting Fit and Lean with Exercise

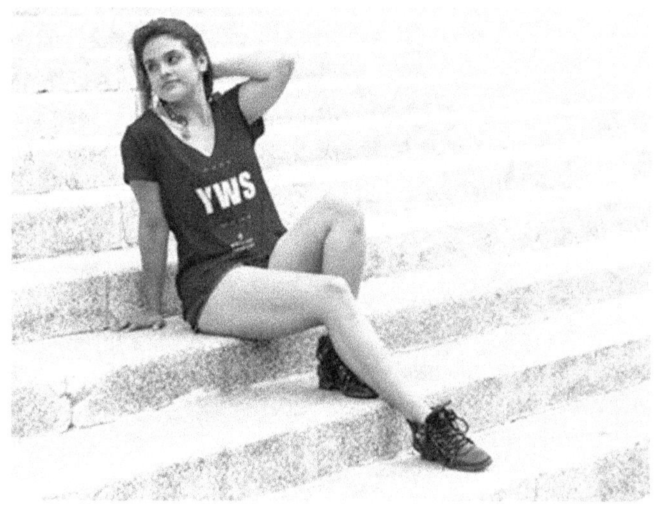

For many of us even the mere mention of the word 'exercise' causes us to cringe and slither away in resignation and if that accurately describes you that is ok because there is hope. Unfortunately, many of us feel that way because we have been wrongly conditioned to think that exercising has to be strenuous and unbearable in order to be effective but that is simply not true. The key to getting anything done is to start (and while this is easier said than done, you have to get up and get going).

If you are in the habit of procrastinating, then you should consider the following Japanese method called 'Kaizen' that is used overcome the practice of putting things off or failing to get things done. According to the 'Kaizen' ideology, if you are required to do something that you are not keen on doing (such as exercising in this instance) then you should do it for a single minute at the same time every day until you get into the habit of doing it. So now that we have given you a way to get off the couch let us guide you into getting it done. Come on, you can do it!

Exercising for good health has many benefits as it helps to prevent heart disease, high blood pressure, lowers your cholesterol and helps you to lose weight. Activities like riding a bike, hiking, walking, or even dancing will help you burn excess fat and get you on the path to a healthy and active lifestyle. Choosing an exercise program should have realistic objectives and it should be accompanied by a meal plan that is sensible and not one that will leave you starving.

Always start slow and with a low-level of intensity and try to monitor your progress over time and slowly increase the intensity level if needed. Should you start your exercise regimen aggressively, you may end up injuring yourself and this may prevent you from engaging in any physical activity thus hindering you from achieving your goal. A good rule of the thumb is to warm up by doing some stretching, taking a 10-15 minute walk, or getting on an elliptical before attempting to do any type of exercises or workout.

If you are not sure how much exercise is required to maintain a healthy lifestyle, the recommendation is about 30-60 minutes of low to moderate intensity, which walking, biking, hiking, and dancing will take care of. If you prefer to exercise in the comfort and privacy of your home and forego any membership fees and noise at a local fitness gym, you can do calisthenics such as sit-ups, lunges, squats, push-ups. Using your own weight for resistance is not only ideal for this type of exercise; but it can also give you results and save you time.

As you progress and improve your physical condition, you may want to consider joining soccer, softball or some shinny hockey league. Whatever you choose, the idea is to keep and remain active and gradually increase the intensity level. Ensure you get plenty of rest and get the recommended daily intake of proper foods and water to keep your metabolism going.

Once you have attained a certain fitness level and feel you need more challenging exercises, you may want to look into buying a treadmill or resistance bands and free weights (dumbbells) which are very inexpensive, but that is entirely up to you and your financial situation. Be sure to mix up your exercises by adding variety to your program and in so doing this will confuse the body and keep the fat-burning process going.

By keeping active and eating sensibly, you can avoid unnecessary weight gain. Patience is a virtue and with repetition, this will definitely help you to develop a new and healthy habit for the rest of your life. However, it is very important that you see your doctor before you begin an exercise or any weight loss program.

Very Simple Tips To Get A Fit Body

Anyone who has ever tried their hand at a fitness program knows the inherent difficulties and obstacles that can and will stand in their way. Fitness is a challenge but don't be discouraged. It is something that with the right discipline and motivation anyone achieve. Here are a few tips to help you in your pursuit of a good body:

- Don't let injuries stop you from exercising. For example, if you hurt your leg, do not stop, continue your workout out on the other leg. Studies have shown that when strengthening one limb alone, the other limb actually increases strength as well so do not let an injury be an excuse not to workout.
- If you are aiming to build muscle, you must eat immediately following your workout because, after you weight train, your muscles breakdown. This is the time your muscles need nutrients the most in order to repair themselves. If you do not feed your muscles immediately after a workout, you could actually experience muscle loss!
- If you want your kids to get more exercise, try making it a competition. Buy everyone in your family a pedometer. Each day marks down how many steps each person has walked. At the end of the week, tally the totals up and see

who the winner is. Come up with a good prize for the winner - a new toy, an extra dessert, or getting to choose dinner for the night.

- You'll burn more calories standing than sitting. Stand while talking on the phone. Better yet, try a standing desk or improvise with a high table or counter. Eat lunch standing up. Trade instant messaging and phone calls for walks to other desks or offices. There are many ways you can find to burn calories while at work.

- It's always a good idea to work out with a partner. This is because they will give you motivation to actually go to the gym regularly. It is also important to bring them because they will spot you on things like a bench press so you do not end up hurting yourself.

- A simple way to improve overall fitness can be done right at home. Whenever an individual is at home they can go up and down the stairs an extra time for every time they use the stairs. By doing this one will double the amount of exercise that they would get from using the stairs.

- If you find yourself exercising infrequently, or making excuses to avoid exercise, make a schedule. Plan on working out a set number of days per week, and keep to your schedule no matter what. If you absolutely must miss a day of fitness, schedule a makeup day and treat it with equal importance.

- Cooling down after a work out will help stop some of the muscle soreness caused by lactic acid build-up, but, you can also try massage. Massage will also work to help your recovery from your gym sessions. A massage is also a great reward for all of your hard work.

- You should always hold your stretches. It does not matter your age, if you are not holding the stretch for at least thirty seconds, you are not maintaining your flexibility. The older you get, the longer you need to hold the pose to achieve the same result. Add thirty additional seconds if you are over forty.

- Alternative sports can offer people good fitness options for people, alongside the more regular forms of exercise.

Free- running is a sport that emphasizes full-body fitness. Climbing, running, and general agility are the main requirements to free- run as you run, climb, and jump across many obstacles. Not only are they fun, but they also unleash your inner child's desire to run and jump over railings, off the beaten path of adulthood.

In order to be successful in increasing your health and fitness level, you have to begin with a plan. Use the ideas you have just read to formulate a plan and start on the road to health and fitness. Do not be discouraged if you don't immediately know where to begin, these tips will get you on your way.

Debunking The Myths

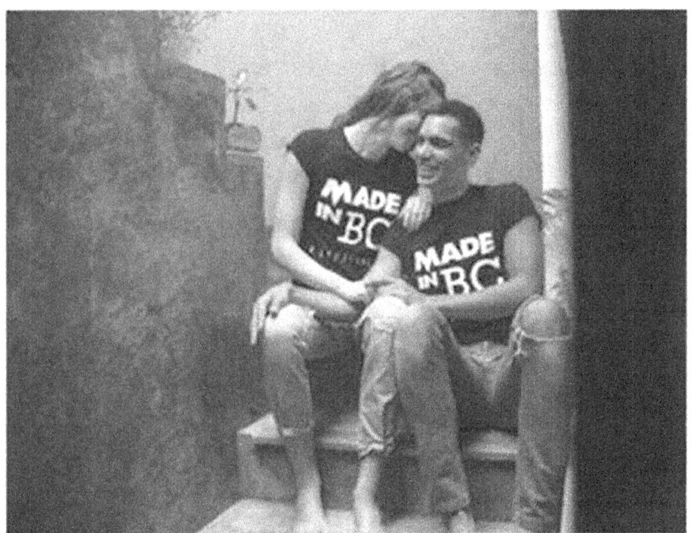

The Lies and Excuses that Rob us of the Ability to Live a Healthy Lifestyle:

I have to exercise a lot.
This is not true.

Actually, I should clarify. It depends on what you call "a lot." If 30 minutes daily or at least 6 times a week is " a lot", then maybe yes. However, you do not always have to do structured exercises- such as going to the gym, lifting weights, or doing cardio. It can be a usual activity, for instance, taking the dog for a walk, throwing a football, playing frisbee, whatever. The most important thing is to get off your butt and move. Don't sit when you can stand, don't stand when you can walk. Get up and walk around the house or office every 20-30 minutes. Go window shopping. Clean the house. Cleaning the house can easily burn 200-300 calories-

depending on the size of the house and exactly what you do, of course.

I have to eat 6 times a day.
Nope. You can if you want to, but you don't have to. Research has shown that an isocaloric diet (same amount of calories and composition) shows no "metabolic advantage" as far as calorie burn goes, to eating more often. You don't have to "stoke the metabolic fire." Some people find that they feel better eating smaller meals more often. Others like a few larger meals. Some like meals and small snacks, the key is to eat healthy. So go ahead and have it! Whatever will help you eat consistently well, and fits into your lifestyle, is what you should do.

I don't have time to exercise.
Really? Now, this is not going to win me any fans, but would you ever say you don't have time to brush your teeth? Take a shower? You find time to do the things that are important to you. We all have the same 24 hours in a day, we all have responsibilities and things we have to do. If something is important,you figure it out and make it happen. If someone said they'd give you a million dollars if you exercised, I bet you'd find a way to get it done. And again it doesn't have to be organized exercise, although it can be. If early in the morning, before the day gets crazy, before the kids/husband/wife/significant other/dog gets up is the only time to exercise, do it! If you can get out at lunchtime, then by all means...!

I don't have time to cook.
Cooking can be much less expensive, as well as much better for you. If you shop smart, buy sale items, stock up, you can eat healthily for a reasonable expenditure. You can also cook large amounts of staple items so you have good food ready to go. And like we said-you make time for what is important to you.

People that are fit are just lucky/genetically gifted/freaks of nature.
This, personally, drives me insane. If someone says to me,"You're so lucky", I tell them,"Actually, luck has nothing to do with it.

Time, consistency, and a lot a hard work and good nutrition do." Yes, we all have different and unique genetics. However, that does not limit you from becoming the healthiest and fittest person you can be. If you have concerns, see your doctor to rule out health issues. Then get moving!

I don't want to get bulky.
This comes from women. I promise you, you will not get bulky. You can, but it would be very intentional, and wouldn't happen overnight, and may require exogenous hormones. I hate to say it, but what many people refer to as "bulky" is most of the time just fat. If you got leaner, you wouldn't think you had too much muscle on your thighs anymore, I can almost guarantee it. When fat covers muscle, that is when the perception of being bulky occurs. For the most part, that is. There are very few women who are genetically blessed to put on muscle easily.

I don't like healthy food.
Nobody really likes boiled chicken and broccoli. However, that is not what you have to eat. You do not have to suffer to lose weight and/or get fit/be healthy. There's a big wide world of food variety to try out! You can add flavor to foods with spices, herbs, citrus, marinades, rubs, various preparation methods-the world is your oyster (or clam, or shrimp, or salmon-get it?) Branch out, read food magazines or sites, wander around the farmers market or grocery store and try something new. There's a ton of wonderful resources and many food blogs that supply recipes that are specifically gluten-free. If you see a recipe you like, take a look and see how it can be modified, if necessary, to meet your nutrition goals. After you do this a few times, it becomes very easy and second nature. I get ideas from the Food Network and then modify as needed for a gluten-free and healthy diet. There's no reason for you to eat anything you don't like. You have many options.

I can't live without (chocolate ice cream, bacon, deep fried onions, candy etc.)
You don't have to. Just make it an indulgence, but just that-an occasional indulgence. Set aside a Saturday dinner to eat what you

want or what you've been craving. When you've been eating well all week, you can have that bit of indulgence with no guilt and no repercussions. If you haven't been eating well all week, then you may want to reconsider. Figure if you eat well 80-90% of the time, take that remaining percentage and have a little bit of an indulgence. That doesn't mean a whole bag of Pamela's Chocolate Chip Simplebites (been there.) Have a few, enjoy them, put them away. In the freezer if necessary. Then enjoy your poison guilt-free again the following week.

I have to get in shape before I start going to the gym.

Nope, just go. No one there cares, they are all too busy worrying about themselves. Just start, give yourself permission to begin. I am always inspired to see people who are new to exercise and the gym, or who are coming back from a layoff. It takes a big decision to make that first step. Little bits at a time, but start. Just begin. Preferably today. Go for a walk. This booklet will be here when you get back.

It's too hard.
Well, I'm not going to lie, it's not easy. But what is harder-making a change, or staying the way you are? Would you prefer to risk getting a chronic lifestyle disease or dying earlier than to do 30 minutes of exercise per day? Changing behavior first requires a change in perspective. Are you truly satisfied and content with your current health and fitness status, your appearance and weight? If so, then that's awesome-stay the same. If not, make a change. Choosing to make a change is probably the hardest part. Actually taking the first few steps to change is pretty hard too. But then it's like a snowball effect-you start to feel/look better, you have more energy, so you want to do more to improve your life. Inertia is a very powerful force but you have the power to overcome it.

Spice Up Your Life - Get Fit and Stay Fit

As with most aspects of our lives, going to the gym can become pretty formulaic pretty quickly and once it becomes routine it generally loses its appeal. Nevertheless, If you're stuck in a workout rut, follow these top five tips to reinvigorate your fitness regime. Bear in mind that finding a new schedule to keep you active needn't just be consigned to a New Year's resolution list but does require a certain amount of discipline, not just to get started but to make it a lifestyle practice.

1. Find a Friend

Working out with a friend is one of the best ways to stick to a workout regime, a consistent friend will ensure that you go to the gym when you say you will. Not only will this keep you on schedule, but there is a competitive element too - watching what someone else does and trying to keep up can be a fantastic motivator, not to mention a welcome distraction as you pound the cross trainer.

2. Classes

Most gyms now provide a schedule for fitness classes. They are well worth joining. The group element provides a real lift, getting you through routines you might think are beyond you, and they push you to go the extra mile. There are lots of interesting classes out there now - it's not just Jane Fonda-style aerobics - so think about Pilates, Zumba, aerobics... the choices are endless and there's something for everyone.

3. Personal Training

Many people avoid personal training like the plague largely because of the cost. One way around this is to hook up with a friend and ask to be trained as a pair. A friend there with you will help you through the session, and halves the cost, giving you all the benefits of one-to-one attention without the huge outlay.

4. Do something new

Whether it's a 10km run for charity, learning to windsurf, or trying a new machine, resolve to do something new every month. When we get into a rut, it affects our minds - we get bored - but in fitness terms, if you don't change your workout regularly you will plateau. Trying something new is good for your mind and body. You may also try adding music to workout and try exercising to unfamiliar but upbeat genres.

5. Think positively

It's easy to slip into the habit of thinking of exercise as a chore. It's not - it's an investment in your future. A healthy body isn't just for twenty- somethings, it's vital for all of us, at every age and stage. Giving yourself the best chance for a long and happy life is something we should all be doing.

Getting fit should be a goal for everyone, not just the sportsmen/sportswomen amongst us. Unfortunately, most people find it difficult to get fit and often don't really know where to start in terms of carrying out the actual exercise. Below are 7 tips to get started on your workout fast and safely.

7 Tips To Get Fit Fast and Safely.

1. Know your limits:

Before embarking on any exercise or diet you should know your limits. This may involve a trip to the doctor's for a check-up and advice and in fact, you should check with your doctor before embarking on any exercise or diet program.

2. Warm up slowly:

This is a very important step that most people don't take seriously. You need to warm up slowly in order to avoid injury. Not only that, you will find the main exercise easier if you have warmed up prior to it.

3. Keep a diary of your diet:

You probably don't actually realize how much you eat. Keep a diet diary and check how many calories you are taking in. It doesn't need to be an in-depth analysis, just an overview of the number of calories you are eating.

4. Keep a diary of your exercise:

Yes, I realize this is the same as the previous point but the key to staying healthy or losing weight is to burn off more calories than you are taking in. It's that simple!

5. Be patient:

You won't get fit in 24hrs. If that is your plan then you are in for a big disappointment. Losing weight takes time and fitness should be a long- term plan that lasts a lifetime.

6. Build up gradually:

Even pro athletes build up their stamina gradually. You won't be running marathons within a week. Build up your exercise gradually and just make sure you are making progress. Even an extra 20 meters is progress when jogging.

7. Variety is the spice of life:

Vary your exercise and diet so you don't get bored. Routine is boring and if exercise is boring you won't stick to it. Vary between walking jogging, cycling, swimming, dancing and television work out especially since the internet is currently replete with them.

Get Healthier Now

Do You Want to Get Healthy Now?

Over the past year, I have focused on improving my health and fitness. Every day is a work in progress for me. By no means am I a health guru or a certified trainer. However, I have made various changes throughout the past year that have given me great results for both my body and mind. I am going to share things that I do and hopefully, they will work for you too.

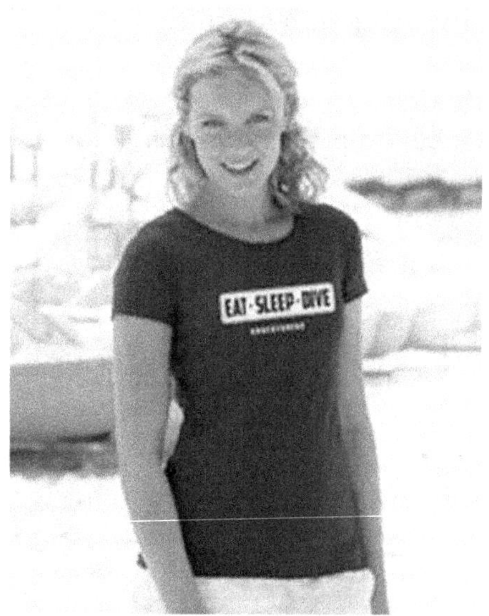

There are several ways for you to get healthy now! Don't think that you have to get it all correct now. Making a major change in your life takes time.

1) Incorporate Fresh Fruits and Vegetables into your Diet Daily
It is important to eat raw foods every day. Adults are

recommended to get between 3 - 6 cups of fruits and vegetables daily. Also, I suggest organic produce whenever it can fit into your budget. If you live anywhere near a farmer's market, get your produce there! Farmer's markets typically have cheaper prices and better quality produce.

2) Exercise Daily

I know you are thinking, "Yeah right who has time to exercise daily?" I do not mean going to the gym and working out for two hours per day, but getting at least 15 mins per day of physical activity. That could simply be taking a quick walk around your neighborhood. It all depends on the results you are looking for. If you want to lose weight, then you should be doing at least three days per week of rigorous physical activity. Know what you want and plan from there.

3) Reduce Processed Foods

If you really want to get healthy now, reduce your intake of processed foods. Processed foods are one of the biggest contributors to weight gain. If you need more validation on this topic, research the mice and McDonald's study. Overall, any name brand food that you eat, there is an organic or natural equivalent in the market. For example, I have replaced all of my son's snacks, the Cheeze-Its, Pop-Tarts, Oreos, Goldfish, with healthier equivalents. They all taste the same or better and he does not even know the difference. You know there is something wrong when there are 20 ingredients listed for a product that normally takes 5 to make it. Good alternative brands to look for are Back to Nature, Cascadian Farm and Annie's for your kid's snacks.

4) Start with a Cleanse

If you want to jump-start your process to get healthy now, try a detox. Detoxes are a great process to remove toxins from your body. Toxins enter into our bodies from the unnatural foods we eat, pollutants in the air outside and chemicals around our homes. There are several ways to detox. I would suggest that you do your research and find a good system that will work for your body and your needs. I like to do a juice cleanse. I will either do a two-day or three day-cleanse. If you have Arden's Garden near you, then I would suggest using their already made detox juice for your first time. Detoxes will make the process to get healthy now, more effective. You may also consider a colon cleanse whether in the form of an enema or colonics to set you off to a clean start.

I hope that you have found these tips on how to get healthy, useful. Remember it is a process. Do not feel like you have to wake up tomorrow and become a vegan. Determine why you want to make the changes to get healthy now and what do you want to get out of the process. Then find the necessary steps to get you there. Pick one strategy at a time; you can start with cutting out processed foods and cut out or reduce your consumption of a different processed food per week or gradually over a month.

A Summary Guide to Healthy Living

1. What is a HEALTHY LIFESTYLE?

A way of living that LOWERS THE RISK of being seriously ill or dying early. Not all illness and disease is preventable; however, some, particularly those along the lines of coronary heart disease and lung cancer can be prevented. Scientific studies have identified certain types of behavior that contribute to serious illness and early death. This booklet aims to help you change your behavior and IMPROVE YOUR HEALTH so that you and your family live longer, healthier lives.

2. What is a HEALTHY LIFESTYLE?

A way of living that HELPS YOU ENJOY more aspects of your life. Health is not just about avoiding a disease or illness. It is about physical, mental and social well-being too. This booklet aims to help you decide to make healthier choices in your lifestyle which will give you more opportunity to ENJOY MORE ASPECTS OF YOUR LIFE FOR LONGER.

3. What are the benefits of a HEALTHY LIFESTYLE?

A way of living that HELPS YOUR WHOLE FAMILY. When you adopt a healthy lifestyle you become a more positive role model for other people in your family, particularly children. You will also create a better environment for them to grow up in. By helping them to follow a healthier lifestyle you will be contributing to their well-being and enjoyment of life now and in the future.

TOBACCO

Smoking is the greatest single self-imposed risk to the health of all. RISKS TO YOU: Respiratory illness, coronary heart disease, cancer RISKS TO YOUR FAMILY: Respiratory illness, chest, nose, ear and throat infections. Your family's risks are increased two to three times if you smoke. Babies who are exposed to tobacco smoke at home are at increased risk of sudden infant death. Young children who have one or more parents who smoke are twice as likely to suffer from chest problems in their first year of life. They will have more chest, nose, ear and throat infections than children whose parents do not smoke. They are also more likely to take up smoking themselves later in life. IF YOU ARE PREGNANT you can damage your baby's chances of being healthy by smoking even before the baby is born.

FACT: Tobacco-related diseases not only lead to many premature deaths but also to years of disease and disability. One-half of all people who regularly smoke will be killed by cigarettes, half in middle age and a half in their senior years. If you stop smoking before middle age you will avoid almost all the increased risk that would have otherwise occurred. Even stopping smoking in middle age can lower your risk. If you don't usetobacco DON'T START. If you do use tobacco you can lower your risk by stopping NOW. You will start experiencing the health benefits.

Conclusion

When asked to list some of the things people would generally like to achieve; things like wealth, happiness and longevity tend to rank high on their agenda. However, I am not in the position to make you a millionaire and there is no guarantee that my presence will you make you happy, but I can tell you that living a healthy lifestyle can add years to your life and it will certainly improve the quality of it.

Therefore, it is imperative that you make a conscious effort to stay healthy, eat right, and you will open yourself up to a new world of opportunities! The key is to begin small and gradually it will get easier as you learn to control cravings and unlearn poor habits that your body is used to.

My recommendation is that you begin with a plan. By setting a plan with a goal linked to a realistic timescale, it will make it easier for you to stick to your workout plan and not relent at the slightest challenge. The thought of achieving your targets will drive you to intensify your work out, therefore leading to better results.

Additionally, the internet is replete with information that will prove useful and there are quite a number of forums, blogs and companies that will assist you in your quest to get fit. Nevertheless, caution must be given to those companies only out to sell their products and before using any product, be sure to vigorously search for legitimate resources and save money by accessing free information and programs.

Once you have set yourself out a plan, the next step is creating a roadmap of how you will actualize your plan. Today, there is a plethora of new and innovative ways to get fit. With technology constantly changing, you can now utilize mobile apps, computer games, many tangible fitness devices and even just general household items. With so many choices the decision can be a difficult one, however, follow the advice of industry professionals or have a look at other customer reviews before purchasing your exercise aid.

Complementary to utililitarian programs and apps are popular activities such as Zumba, Yoga and Pilates. In fact, over the over the past few years we have seen an increase in activities that have injected fun into exercises and have demonstrated that exercises can be fun, calming and good for more than just your waistline.

The health benefits of keeping fit are being cited globally, especially with obesity rates becoming a real concern. In fact, Public Health Agency of Canada has indicated that about 64% of adults in Canada (in this instance, individuals over the age of 18) are considered to be either overweight or obese while 30% of Canadian children between the ages of 5-17 are listed as being either overweight or obese. Additionally, the Daily Mail has highlighted that on average the typical person in Britain will consume 38,000 calories and gain up to 6lbs in weight much to the delight of the gym companies that are poised to potentially reap the rewards of the overindulging public.

Therefore, in light of such findings, you owe it to yourself to move away from engaging in a predominantly sedentary lifestyle and start moving. However, this appeal should not merely result in gym enrolment and membership as many persons are currently doing because a a trip to the gym is not enough. Instead, it is necessary to make changes to your diet, your daily activities as well as your mindset in order to shed the pounds as quickly as possible.

Furthermore, bear in mind, that even when you reach your ideal body, health and fitness is for the long-term, so maintaining your health and ideal body will take determination and a commitment in order to yield positive results. Be sure to try out different fitness methods in order to determine the one that is best for you. Interestingly, there is no one size fits all, so you will need to experiment with a number of exercising techniques before finding the one that will yield the best results.

Just always keep in mind that exercising should be fun as well as beneficial, This way you will be more likely to work out and it will last longer than a short-term phase. The next step after looking up a fitness program is research. This can be a very interesting experience... or... a very frustrating one. However, if you are feeling the latter, I am here to help.

Here's the truth in a nutshell: These days, it is hard to tell whether a review is from a genuine user or if it has been generated by the company itself. It appears as if the users of many fitness programs are simply giving rehearsed comments that are strikingly vague and are not proving to be as useful as they should be in influencing decision making.

Similarly, many of the fitness companies are regurgitating existing techniques and are rebranding and are selling them as something new. For a beginner, this can be very confusing because it appears there are so many different approaches to getting fit. (I'm not saying there aren't, but not in the way that these companies are making it out to be.)

In fact, I've come to realize that weight loss and muscle gain techniques haven't changed much in recent history but the way they are being marketed has. Sure, I've learned a couple of different tips from different programs I've investigated over the years but there's never anything too surprising and most of the information given out is always common sense. When it comes down to it there are only a few things you need to do to start getting fit and healthy. In conclusion, there are no shortcuts, just follow these 3 simple instructions to be on the right path today. Here is the fundamental 'Rule of Threes':

Eat well - Without a proper nutritional diet your gym work is for nothing. Re-fuel your body with the good stuff, veg, lean meat, water, fruits, dairy, grains and carbohydrates. I think of it as 70% what you eat and 30% working out. What you eat is so important and I don't think people realize this enough. I recently spoke to someone who asked if they should starve themselves after exercise. I was more than speechless but there are persons who actually do this. I would advise you to eat balanced meals in order to get the energy to exercise.

Exercise effectively - I see so many people at the gym jogging on the treadmill for an hour+. This might be good for endurance training but weight loss?... Start doing interval training or circuit training 3 times a week for 30 minutes and you'll burn twice the amount of calories. Make sure you exercise effectively, it's not just what you do but how you do it. Whether it's performing a rep with good form or using the right trainers on a run.

Drink Water like it is actually going out of fashion - Try and drink 8 pints a day (I know you've heard it before but it is true). After all, we are 70% water and you need to stay hydrated in order to maintain as healthy lifestyle. Here's an interesting bench mark; Pinch the fat around your waist. If it wobbles when you let go then it is more than likely water more water retention than fat. So start drinking the good stuff! You'll see a difference in a couple of days.

So, there you have it but before you sign up for a fancy fitness program, take the leap and follow the steps in this book and see where you get. The main thing that you need is motivation which unfortunately you cannot buy, but you can find the internal drive to push yourself, bearing in mind that I am routing for you! So, get up and get going because you can do it! Good luck!